Manage Your Blood Pressure

Vivek Kamath

ISBN-13:978-1523966950

ACKNOWLEDGEMENT

I am grateful to my mother Late Mrs. Vimala Kamath for giving me the birth because of which I am able to attain this great moment of writing a book on "Manage Your Blood Pressure". My Mother died of Diabetes and Cardiac Aliment way back in November 2006. Today I am able to cure Diabetes, Heart Ailment, blood pressure, Cholesterol and any respiratory diseases thru Reiki healing method and many other diseases without Medicines. It was unfortunate that I do not have my mother with me. I am sure her departed soul will now be able to rest in peace today by seeing the achievement of her beloved son. My mother's love and affection was a key for me to attain this position today and instrumental in shaping up my life and destiny. I am very thankful to my mother for giving me this great opportunity to serve the world.

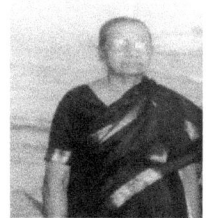

I would like to express my gratitude and heart-full of love to great Reiki Guru and Founder Dr Mikao Usui of Japan.

I would like to thank myself because of my inner strength with which I could able to convert the difficult situations or challenges faced in my life as a great opportunity for learning and always believed that life is a continuous education process. Furthermore, I strongly believed in my life that whatever happens in life it will happen for a good cause and these are based on our good and bad karma/action of past and current life.

CONTENTS

1 Introduction

Background about the Author

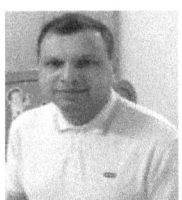

Author Vivek Kamath is an Indian Software Engineer by profession. Author has worked with the world's top International Banks across the globe for nearly 20 years to manage large scale Information Technology (IT) projects. Author is also a Reiki Healing Master Cum Practitioner and Practicing Reiki Healing, Mexican Healing, Crystal Healing, Melchizedek Method of healing from the last 5 years. Author has healed many diabetic patients, blood pressure patients (both high and low blood pressure), Heart Patients (removed the heart blocks), removed kidney stones , cured sinusitis, severe joint pains, constipation, migraines, headaches, insomnia, stomach related problems, diabetic gum problems, skin problems (dry skin, eczema) and chronic nasal allergies, nasal blockages without any medicines. Some of the above treatments have been completed within a week to maximum 1 month duration. Author has intention to help as much as diabetic patients to come out of the disease without any medicines. Author has an intention to build a healing center for diabetic patients across the globe.

For whom was this book prepared?

This book intended for people who are suffering from high blood pressure and low blood pressure. There are various Healing methods to heal blood pressure and heart diseases.. Author has mentioned about the Reiki Healing in this book.

Author has intention to help as much as patients who are suffering from high blood pressure and low blood pressure. Author has cured some low blood pressure patients within 15days of healing. Allopathic medicines has many dangerous side effects and it needs to be taken for a life time. If in case you are not able to heal by yourself, please feel free to contact author directly by email.

Author has healed several of his patients who were having high and low blood pressure and heart ailment problems. All of the patients have been completely cured from these diseases without any medicines. Author has used distant healing method (Patients can reside far away from the healer) of Reiki to heal some of the patients. Distant healing has been found to be very effective.

2 What is Blood Pressure?

Blood is carried from the heart to all parts of our body in vessels called arteries. Blood pressure is the force of the blood pushing against the walls of the arteries. Each time the heart beats (about 60-72 times a minute at rest), it pumps out blood into the arteries.

What is systolic pressure?

Our blood pressure is at its highest when the heart beats, pumping the blood. This is called systolic pressure.

What is diastolic pressure?

When our heart is at rest, between beats, our blood pressure falls. This is the diastolic pressure.

Norma Blood pressure is 120/80 mmHg. The top number is the systolic(120) and the bottom the diastolic(80). Blood pressure changes during the day. It is lowest as you sleep and rises when you get up. It also can rise when you are excited, nervous, or active.

What is high blood pressure?

We probably have high blood pressure (hypertension) if your blood pressure readings are consistently 140 over 90, or higher, over a number of weeks.

We may also have high blood pressure if just one of the numbers is higher than it should be over a number of weeks.

If we have high blood pressure, this higher pressure puts extra strain on your heart and blood vessels. Over time, this extra strain increases your risk of a heart attack or stroke.

High blood pressure can also cause heart and kidney disease, and is closely linked to some forms of dementia.

What is low blood pressure?

It is also called as hypotension. A low blood pressure reading is having a level that is 90/60 mmHg or lower is considered as low blood pressure. If the top number(systolic pressure) is 90 or less (regardless of the bottom number) this may be low blood pressure. Also if the bottom number (diastolic pressure) is 60 or less (regardless of the top number) this may be low blood pressure. The low pressure can make us faint or dizzy.

3. What are the Causes of Blood Pressure?

1. Genetic (Heredity) reason may be one of the cause of high blood pressure
2. Age and Unhealthy life style is also another of the cause of the blood pressure

3. According to some research, some ethnic origin people from African-Caribbean and South Asian communities are at greater risk than other people of high blood pressure.

4. Unhealthy eating habits, excess salt (food with excess sodium) intake, people with vitamin D deficiency, sedentary life style, obesity, excess alcohol consumption, smoking and consuming excess salt in our diet are the key factors impacting the high blood pressure.

5. Some Allopathic medicines or health conditions (kidney disorder, heart ailments and uncontrolled diabetes, uncontrolled thyroid problems and Sleep Apnea) may increase the blood pressure. All 4 major diseases diabetes, high blood pressure, kidney and cardiac disease are inter linked.

6. Stress is the major factor for the high blood pressure

7. There is no specific reasons for low blood pressure. It may be because of some health conditions or medicines can cause to develop low blood pressure.

4. Symptoms of Blood Pressure

Hypertension (High Blood Pressure) is a silent killer because it has no early significant symptoms or signs, but creates an extra load on the heart and blood vessels. The only way to know if we have high blood pressure is to have test it. However, a single high reading does not necessarily mean we have high blood pressure. Many things can affect our blood pressure through the day, so our doctor will take a number of blood pressure readings to see that it stays high over time.

With regard to Hypotension (low blood pressure), there is no allopathic medicines. The signs of low blood pressure are patients may feel faint and dizziness.

5. Complication of Blood Pressure

High blood pressure (hypertension) puts extra strain on your heart and blood vessels. This can cause them to become weaker or damaged.

The higher your blood pressure, the higher your risk of serious health problems as mentioned below.

1. Heart Attack or a stroke

2. Brain Stroke or some forms of dementia

3. It can cause a kidney disease

4. There are possibility it can affect the limbs a peripheral arterial disease.

5. If the patients are already suffering from killer

diabetes or high cholesterol, high blood pressure can jeopardize the existing disease and organs.

6. Test for Blood Pressure

Blood Pressure Test

A sphygmomanometer is the devise used to measure blood pressure.

	Normal Blood Pressure In mm Hg	High Blood Pressure In mm Hg	Low Blood Pressure In mm Hg
Systolic	120	Above 130	90 or below
Diastolic	80	Above 90	60 or below

Please note that for low blood pressure if the systolic reading is 90 or less (regardless of the diastolic reading) this may be low blood pressure. Similarly, if the diastolic pressure is 60 or less (regardless of the systolic pressure) this may be considered as low blood pressure. But, it is advisable to take at least 5 to 7 readings in a span of 2 months to check the accuracy.

7. Facts Findings on Blood Pressure

1. High blood pressure can lead to diseases including heart disease, stroke, vascular dementia and chronic kidney disease

2. Globally, nearly one billion people have high blood pressure (hypertension); of these, two-thirds are in developing countries

3. Hypertension is one of the most important causes of premature death worldwide and the problem is growing; in 2025, an estimated 1.56 billion adults will be living with hypertension

4. Globally 11% of all disease burden and in developed countries are caused by raised blood pressure (hypertension)

5. 50% of CHD (Coronary Heart Disease) and almost 75% of heart strokes in developed countries are attributable to a systolic blood pressure over 115 mmHg.

6. About 70 million Americans—one in three adults—have high blood pressure, but only about half of them have it under control. Recent deaths related to hypertension (HTN) in USA have soared by 61.8 % compared to 2000

7. Projections show that by 2030, ≈41.4% of US adults will have hypertension

8. High blood pressure was a primary or contributing cause of death for more than **360,000 Americans** in 2013—that's nearly **1,000 deaths each day**

9. High blood pressure costs USA nearly **$46 billion** each year

10. In the United Kingdom (UK) over half of the estimated 16 million people living with high blood pressure are unaware they have the condition, as it is symptomless

11. In UK, The number of strokes occurring in men aged between 40 and 54 has rocketed by almost 50% in less than 15 years, according to the Stroke Association U.K

12. High blood pressure is the UK's biggest silent killer, responsible for 60% of strokes and 40% of heart attacks

13. New figures from Public Health England (PHE) reveal that diseases caused by high blood pressure are estimated to cost the NHS over £2 billion every year

14. A total of 26.6% of Chinese adults had hypertension, and a significantly greater number of men were hypertensive than women

15. In India this number is on a steady incline. A recent study revealed that, 200 million Indians suffered from High Blood Pressure

16. People living on the northern islands of Japan eat more salt per capita than anyone else in the world and have the highest incidence of essential hypertension. By contrast, people who add no salt to their food show virtually no traces of essential hypertension

8.Cure for Blood Pressure

There are several methods to cure to high or low blood pressure without medicines.

Below are the some of the healing techniques used across the world to cure blood pressure. I am highlighting only Reiki Healing and Relevant Yoga's and Mudra's to normalize blood pressure.

A. Reiki Healing

B. Crystal Healing

C. Pranic Healing

D. Mexican Healing

E. Holographic Healing

F. Yoga and Mudra

Reiki Healing for Blood Pressure

A.   Reiki Healing

Reiki is a form of alternative medicine developed in 1922 by Japanese Buddhist Dr. Mikao Usui.

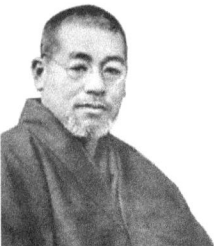

Mikao Usui 臼井甕男(1865–1926)

It uses a technique commonly called palm healing or hands-on-healing.The word Reiki is made of two Japanese words – Rei which means "God's Wisdom or the Higher Power" and Ki which means "life force energy". So Reiki is actually "spiritually guided life force energy or universal energy".

Any blood related disease can be completely healed using Reiki Healing. Distant Healing (Patients need not be present in the physical location of the healer/Reiki Practitioner) method found to be very effective. Our heart governs the blood flowing out and in to the heart and body. In terms of Chakra healing, Reiki healer needs to heal the heart chakra of the patient. Also, healer needs to focus on healing the entire heart if there is a significant high blood pressure or even blood pressure. Healer needs to normalize the systolic and diastolic pressure of the heart.

This healing can cure both high blood pressure and low blood pressure.

With the Reiki, we can set the body clock and timer for removing the negative energies for the life time from the heart's circularly system. By doing this, we can permanently cure any chronic blood related or heart ailments diseases.

Yoga For Blood Pressure

Yoga is a Sanskrit word meaning "union" and is about getting the mind and the body to work together to find balance, harmony and ultimately better health .Yoga is Physical, mental and spiritual practice or discipline which originated in India. Yoga Gurus from India introduced yoga to the western countries.

In 1980's yoga became popular as a system of physical exercise across the western world. Yoga in Indian Traditions, however is more than physical exercise, it has a meditative and spiritual core.

Yoga can help to calm the mind, which is more important than you probably realize. One of the reason for the high blood pressure problem may be a constant source of worry and stress for varying different reasons. Yoga can help you to relax (both mentally and physically) and forget any worries through breathing and meditation.

Yoga moves can specifically help ease heart system related issues. With regular practice, yoga could help to keep your cardiac system working at its best, and prevent any blood related related issues. Below list of yoga's are useful for blood pressure reduction which you can find in Appendix

9. Manage your blood pressure in Nut-Shell

In Nut-shell Below are the Blood Pressure Normalization Summary you may need to keep in mind.

Food Diet

1. Follow the Appendix A and B food to eat and not to eat for High and Low Blood Pressure

2. Always make a habit of drinking 3 Liters of water on daily basis. This will help to release the toxic or negative energies from our body.

3. Reduce your salt in-take in diet, increase potassium in-take in diet (provided you do not have other diseases like Kidney diseases)

4. Reduce Smoking and In-take of Alcohol

Exercise

1. Conduct those Yoga which helps the Cardiac System healing (provided in book please refer to appendix)
2. Ensure you walk every day for 30 to 45 minutes.

Life Style Changes

1. Practice Yoga or Meditation to reduce your stress, depression and anxiety levels

2. Practice some stress management techniques to reduce stress level

3. If you have time, practice 7 Chakra Meditation weekly once

4. Practice Blood Pressure Mudra for 15 minutes daily or thrice a week

5. Practice some deep breathing exercises helps to ease the body circulatory and cardiac systems

6. Practice Reiki Healing on weekly basis helps you to balance all 7 Chakras which keeps you in good mental and physical health

7. Heal your Heart Chakra on regular basis to heal the Cardiac System. If you follow this on regular basis, you will not have any blood pressure . This healing should take care of your any problem related to heart or lungs.

Appendix A Food to be taken to normalize high blood pressure/low blood pressure

	Food	Effectiveness in Reducing High Blood Pressure
1	**Oats**	Fibrous food lowers the absorption of bad cholesterol in the bloodstream. Oats has high fiber content which influences to increase good cholesterol and reduce the high blood pressure.
2	**Wholegrain**	Wholegrain flour has high fiber. Fiber is required to maintain good level of HDL in the blood and reduce the blood pressure. Switch from white bread to whole wheat bread for your breakfast or sandwiches.
3	**Omega 3**	Omega 3 from fishes like salmon, sardines, mackerel and Tuna. Omega 3 not only reduces cholesterol but also helps to reduce high blood pressure.
4	**Flaxseeds, White Beans & Quinoa**	For those who are vegetarian they can opt for Flaxseeds in your dishes or salads. Flaxseeds are rich in fibre and

Omega-3. Flaxseeds are very useful in lowering cholesterol, lower blood pressure, diabetes and heart diseases.

Quinoa – can be used in your diet to reduce the blood pressure level.

5	**Vegetables**	The vegetables like broccoli, potatoes, beet roots and Sweet Potatoes, Red Bell Pepper, Kale and Celery. These veggies have the power to control your blood pressure.
6	**Fruits**	Bananas, pears, guava, grapefruit, avocados, prunes and berries are rich in calcium, antioxidants and fiber, but they can lower your blood pressure,
7	**Indian Gooseberry(Amla)**	This is very effective in reducing blood pressure level. Grate the Amla and make the Juice. Drinking thrice a day can drastically reduce blood pressure level by 80%.
8	**Wheat Grass Juice**	Wheat Grass Juice is highly effective in reducing the blood pressure level.

Appendix B Food to be avoided to maintain to manage good blood pressure

	Type of Food
1	Fried Foods
2	Micro wave Food
3	Shell Fish
4	Red Meat
5	Cheese and Diary Items
6	Ice Creams
7	Fast Foods
8	Energy Drinks
9	White Rice, Breads, pastries, pasta made of white flour
10	Canned Food

Appendix C Yoga for Blood Pressure

I have not documented how to perform these yoga steps in this book. I would advise readers to check with your professional yoga teacher and perform these yoga's under their guidance. You can perform any few Yoga poses from the below list. Asana is nothing but pose.

1. Sukhasan
2. Paschimottanasana
3. Purvatanuasana
4. Shvasana
5. Ardh-halasana
6. Setu Bandhasana
7. Makarasana
8. Shishuasana
9. Vajrasana
10. Suptvajrasana

Appendix D Mudra Blood Pressure

Please note the below mudra's for high and low blood pressure.

For High Blood Pressure

1. Vaayan Mudra

2. Aakash Mudra

3. Pitta-naashak Mudra

4. Apaan- Vaayu Mudra

For Low Blood Pressure

1. Prithvi vardhak Mudra

2. Aakash-shaamak Mudra

www.ingramcontent.com/pod-product-compliance
Lightning Source LLC
Chambersburg PA
CBHW072030280526
45788CB00007B/2740